Title:

The Path to Vitality: HEALTH IS NEW WELATH

AUTHOR   ZOHAIB HASSAN KHAN

"Health is not just about the absence of illness; it's the vibrant energy that fuels our dreams, the resilient spirit that conquers challenges, and the boundless vitality that propels us toward our fullest potential."

Are you ready to embark on a journey to unlock the secrets to a vibrant, fulfilling life? Imagine waking up each day feeling energized, resilient, and ready to seize the opportunities that life has to offer. In "The Vitality Code," you'll discover a transformative guide to achieving lifelong health, happiness, and vitality like never before.

Through captivating storytelling, expert insights, and actionable advice, this book takes you on a riveting exploration of what it truly means to thrive in every aspect of your life. From nourishing your body with delicious, nutrient-rich foods to cultivating mindfulness, resilience, and meaningful connections, each chapter is packed with practical strategies and empowering wisdom to help you live your best life.

Delve into the science of optimal health and well-being as you uncover the power of nutrition, exercise, and stress management to fuel your vitality. Learn how to harness the transformative benefits of mindfulness and gratitude to cultivate joy, presence, and inner peace in your daily life. Explore the profound connection between physical health, emotional well-being, and spiritual fulfillment as you embark on a journey of self-discovery and personal growth.

Whether you're seeking to revitalize your energy, boost your immune system, or simply enhance your overall quality of life, "The Vitality Code" offers a roadmap to success that's both inspiring and practical. With its engaging narrative, captivating insights, and actionable strategies, this book will empower you to take control of your health, happiness, and vitality like never before.

Prepare to be amazed as you unlock the secrets to lifelong vitality and embark on a journey of transformation that will leave you feeling invigorated, empowered, and inspired. "The Vitality Code" is more than just a book—it's your passport to a life filled with health, happiness, and boundless vitality. Are you ready to unlock your full potential and live your best life? Dive into "The Vitality Code" today and discover the power of thriving in every aspect of your life.

TABLE OF CONTENT

Introduction:

Introduce the importance of living a healthy lifestyle.

Explain the purpose and structure of the book.

Understanding Health:

Define what health means and why it's important.

Discuss the interconnectedness of physical, mental, and emotional health.

Nutrition and Diet:

Explore the principles of a balanced diet.

Discuss the importance of macronutrients, micronutrients, and hydration.

Provide practical tips for healthy eating and meal planning.

Exercise and Fitness:

Explain the benefits of regular physical activity.

Discuss different types of exercise and their effects on the body.

Offer guidance on creating a personalized fitness plan.

Sleep and Rest:

Explain the importance of sleep for overall health and well-being.

Discuss common sleep problems and how to address them.

Provide tips for improving sleep quality and establishing healthy sleep habits.

Stress Management:

Explore the impact of stress on health.

Discuss effective stress management techniques such as mindfulness, meditation, and relaxation exercises.

Provide strategies for managing stress in everyday life.

Social Connections and Relationships:

Discuss the importance of social support for health and well-being.

Explore ways to build and maintain meaningful relationships.

Offer tips for improving communication and conflict resolution in relationships.

Mental Stimulation and Cognitive Health:

Discuss the importance of mental stimulation for brain health.

Explore activities that promote cognitive function and prevent cognitive decline.

Provide tips for maintaining mental sharpness and cognitive agility.

Avoiding Harmful Substances:

Discuss the health risks associated with tobacco, alcohol, and drug use.

Offer strategies for reducing or eliminating harmful substances from your life.

Provide resources for seeking help with addiction or substance abuse.

Creating a Healthy Lifestyle:

Summarize key principles for living a healthy life.

Offer practical advice for integrating healthy habits into daily life.

Provide encouragement and motivation for readers to prioritize their health and well-being.

Conclusion:

Recap the main points of the book.

Encourage readers to take action and make positive changes in their lives.

Offer additional resources for further exploration and support.

Chapter 1: ***The Foundation of Health***

We all know that a balanced diet, regular exercise, and sufficient sleep are important for our health, but have you ever wondered why? In this chapter, we'll explore the science behind these fundamental aspects of well-being and how they contribute to our vitality.

- Understanding the importance of a balanced diet: What does it mean to eat a balanced diet, and how does it benefit our bodies? We'll delve into the role of macronutrients like carbohydrates, proteins, and fats, as well as the importance of micronutrients such as vitamins and minerals. We'll also discuss the impact of diet on energy levels, mood, and overall health.
- The role of hydration and its impact on overall well-being: We often hear that we should drink plenty of water, but what does adequate hydration really do for us? We'll explore the benefits of staying well-hydrated, from supporting digestion and circulation to promoting clear skin and cognitive function.
- Exploring the connection between mental and physical health: How are our mental and physical health interconnected? We'll discuss the ways in which stress, emotions, and mental well-being can influence our physical health, and vice versa. Understanding this connection is crucial for achieving holistic vitality.

Understanding the Importance of a Balanced Diet

Introduction to Nutrition:

Define the concept of nutrition and its significance in maintaining overall health.

Discuss the essential nutrients required by the body, including macronutrients (carbohydrates, proteins, and fats) and micronutrients (vitamins and minerals).

Principles of a Balanced Diet:

Explain what constitutes a balanced diet, emphasizing the importance of variety, moderation, and portion control.

Discuss the role of each macronutrient and micronutrient in supporting different bodily functions.

Health Benefits of a Balanced Diet:

Explore the numerous health benefits associated with consuming a balanced diet, such as weight management, improved energy levels, better mood regulation, and reduced risk of chronic diseases.

Provide examples of specific foods that contribute to overall health and well-being.

Practical Tips for Healthy Eating:

Offer practical advice on how to incorporate more nutritious foods into daily meals and snacks.

Discuss strategies for meal planning, grocery shopping, and preparing healthy meals on a budget.

Provide guidance on navigating food labels and making informed choices when dining out.

The Role of Hydration and Its Impact on Overall Well-being

Understanding Hydration:

Explain the importance of hydration for maintaining proper bodily functions, including temperature regulation, nutrient transportation, and waste removal.

Discuss the body's water needs and factors that influence hydration levels, such as age, activity level, and environmental conditions.

Health Benefits of Proper Hydration:

Explore the various health benefits associated with staying adequately hydrated, such as improved cognitive function, better athletic performance, and enhanced skin health.

Discuss the role of hydration in preventing common health problems like constipation, urinary tract infections, and kidney stones.

Signs of Dehydration and Overhydration:

Identify the signs and symptoms of dehydration and overhydration, emphasizing the importance of listening to the body's thirst cues.

Provide guidance on how to recognize when to increase fluid intake and when to seek medical attention for hydration-related issues.

Tips for Staying Hydrated:

Offer practical tips for maintaining proper hydration throughout the day, such as carrying a reusable water bottle, flavoring water with fruits and herbs, and consuming hydrating foods like fruits and vegetables.

Exploring the Connection Between Mental and Physical Health

Understanding Mental Health:

Define mental health and explain its significance in overall well-being.

Discuss the interconnectedness of mental and physical health, highlighting how one can influence the other.

Impact of Mental Health on Physical Health:

Explore the ways in which mental health conditions, such as stress, anxiety, and depression, can affect physical health outcomes, including immune function, cardiovascular health, and sleep quality.

Discuss the concept of psychosomatic illness and how mental stressors can manifest as physical symptoms.

Impact of Physical Health on Mental Health:

Discuss how physical activity, nutrition, sleep, and other lifestyle factors can positively impact mental health outcomes, such as mood regulation, stress management, and cognitive function.

Provide examples of exercise modalities and dietary patterns that have been shown to support mental well-being.

Practical Strategies for Enhancing Mental and Physical Health:

Offer practical strategies for promoting holistic health, emphasizing the importance of self-care practices, social support networks, and seeking professional help when needed.

Provide resources for accessing mental health services and support groups for individuals struggling with mental health issues.

By exploring these topics in depth, readers can gain a comprehensive understanding of the foundation of health and learn practical strategies for improving their overall well-being.

Chapter 2: *Nourishing Your Body*

Introduction to Nourishment:

Define nourishment as the process of providing the body with essential nutrients for growth, repair, and maintenance.

Discuss the significance of nourishing the body with wholesome foods for optimal health and well-being.

The Importance of Nutrient-Dense Foods:

Explain the concept of nutrient density, which refers to foods that provide a high concentration of essential nutrients relative to their caloric content.

Emphasize the benefits of prioritizing nutrient-dense foods such as fruits, vegetables, whole grains, lean proteins, and healthy fats in the diet.

Key Nutrients for Health and Vitality:

Explore essential nutrients necessary for optimal health, including vitamins, minerals, protein, carbohydrates, and fats.

Discuss the roles of these nutrients in supporting various bodily functions and overall well-being.

Creating Balanced Meals and Snacks:

Provide guidance on building balanced meals that incorporate a variety of nutrient-dense foods from different food groups.

Offer practical tips for meal planning, portion control, and incorporating healthy snacks to maintain energy levels throughout the day.

Eating for Energy and Performance:

Discuss the importance of fueling the body with the right nutrients to support physical activity, mental focus, and overall performance.

Provide recommendations for pre- and post-workout nutrition to optimize energy levels, hydration, and recovery.

Mindful Eating Practices:

Introduce the concept of mindful eating, which involves paying attention to hunger and fullness cues, savoring flavors and textures, and practicing gratitude for nourishing food.

Offer strategies for cultivating mindful eating habits, such as eating slowly, minimizing distractions, and practicing gratitude.

Addressing Dietary Preferences and Restrictions:

Acknowledge that dietary preferences, allergies, intolerances, and cultural considerations can impact food choices and eating habits.

Provide guidance on how to adapt dietary patterns to accommodate individual needs while still prioritizing nutrient-rich foods.

Navigating Food Marketing and Labels:

Discuss common pitfalls of food marketing, such as misleading health claims and exaggerated nutrition information.

Offer tips for deciphering food labels and making informed choices when selecting packaged foods.

Practical Recipes and Meal Ideas:

Include a selection of simple, nutritious recipes and meal ideas that readers can incorporate into their daily routines.

Provide options for breakfast, lunch, dinner, snacks, and beverages that showcase the diversity and deliciousness of nutrient-dense foods.

Conclusion: Empowering Nourishing Habits:

Summarize the key principles of nourishing the body with nutrient-dense foods.

Encourage readers to prioritize whole, minimally processed foods in their diet and experiment with new ingredients and recipes to support their health and vitality.

Now that we understand the foundational principles of health, let's delve into the specifics of nourishing our bodies with the right foods.

- The benefits of whole foods and the dangers of processed foods: What exactly are whole foods, and why are they superior to processed foods? We'll explore the nutritional value of whole, unprocessed foods and the potential risks associated with consuming heavily processed products.
- The Benefits of Whole Foods and the Dangers of Processed Foods
- Introduction to Whole Foods and Processed Foods:
-
- Define whole foods as minimally processed or unprocessed foods that retain their natural nutrients and fiber, such as fruits, vegetables, whole grains, nuts, and seeds.

- Define processed foods as foods that have undergone significant alterations through manufacturing processes, often containing added sugars, unhealthy fats, sodium, and artificial additives.
- Nutrient Density of Whole Foods:
-
- Explain how whole foods are rich in essential nutrients, including vitamins, minerals, antioxidants, and dietary fiber, which are crucial for supporting overall health and vitality.
- Provide examples of nutrient-dense whole foods and their health benefits, such as leafy greens, berries, quinoa, and wild-caught fish.
- Health Benefits of Whole Foods:
-
- Discuss the numerous health benefits associated with consuming a diet rich in whole foods, including reduced risk of chronic diseases such as heart disease, type 2 diabetes, obesity, and certain cancers.
- Highlight the role of whole foods in promoting satiety, weight management, digestive health, and improved energy levels.
- Processing and Nutrient Loss:
-
- Explain how processing techniques such as refining, milling, and cooking can lead to the loss of essential nutrients, including vitamins, minerals, and fiber, in processed foods.
- Discuss the impact of industrial processing on the nutritional quality of foods and its potential implications for health.
- Additives and Preservatives in Processed Foods:
-

- Explore the use of additives, preservatives, flavor enhancers, and artificial sweeteners in processed foods to improve taste, texture, and shelf life.
- Discuss the potential health risks associated with consuming these additives, including allergic reactions, gastrointestinal issues, and long-term health consequences.
- High Sugar, Salt, and Unhealthy Fat Content:
-
- Highlight the high sugar, salt, and unhealthy fat content found in many processed foods, which can contribute to weight gain, inflammation, insulin resistance, and metabolic disorders.
- Discuss the hidden sources of added sugars, sodium, and trans fats in processed foods and their impact on overall health.
- Impact on Chronic Disease Risk:
-
- Review epidemiological studies linking the consumption of processed foods with an increased risk of obesity, cardiovascular disease, hypertension, dyslipidemia, and other chronic health conditions.
- Discuss the role of processed foods in promoting inflammation, oxidative stress, insulin resistance, and dysbiosis in the gut microbiota.
- Practical Tips for Choosing Whole Foods:
-
- Provide practical tips for incorporating more whole foods into the diet, such as shopping the perimeter of the grocery store, choosing fresh, seasonal produce, and preparing meals from scratch at home.
- Offer guidance on reading food labels, avoiding processed foods with long ingredient lists and unfamiliar additives, and opting for minimally processed alternatives whenever possible.

- Conclusion: Making Informed Food Choices:
-
- Emphasize the importance of prioritizing whole foods over processed foods for optimal health and well-being.
- Encourage readers to become more mindful of their food choices, to focus on quality over quantity, and to embrace a diet rich in nutrient-dense whole foods as a foundation for lifelong health.
-
- The power of superfoods and their impact on vitality: We've all heard about the wonders of superfoods, but what makes them so special? We'll take a closer look at the nutrient-dense qualities of superfoods like berries, leafy greens, and nuts, and how they can contribute to our overall vitality.
- The Power of Superfoods and Their Impact on Vitality
- Introduction to Superfoods:
-
- Define superfoods as nutrient-rich foods that are particularly beneficial for health and well-being due to their high concentrations of vitamins, minerals, antioxidants, and phytochemicals.
- Discuss the growing interest in superfoods and their potential to support vitality and longevity.
- Nutrient Density of Superfoods:
-
- Highlight the exceptional nutrient density of superfoods, which often contain higher levels of essential nutrients compared to other foods.
- Provide examples of common superfoods, such as berries, leafy greens, nuts, seeds, fatty fish, and certain herbs and spices.
- Health Benefits of Superfoods:
-

- Explore the wide range of health benefits associated with consuming superfoods, including enhanced immune function, improved cardiovascular health, reduced inflammation, and increased energy levels.
- Discuss the role of antioxidants in superfoods in combating oxidative stress, protecting cells from damage, and reducing the risk of chronic diseases.
- Specific Superfoods and Their Benefits:
-
- Highlight the health benefits of specific superfoods and their unique nutritional properties. For example:
- Berries: Rich in antioxidants, fiber, and vitamins, berries have been associated with improved cognitive function, reduced inflammation, and lower risk of chronic diseases.
- Leafy Greens: Packed with vitamins, minerals, and phytonutrients, leafy greens like kale, spinach, and Swiss chard support bone health, cardiovascular health, and detoxification.
- Fatty Fish: High in omega-3 fatty acids, fatty fish such as salmon, mackerel, and sardines promote heart health, brain function, and mood regulation.
- Nuts and Seeds: Loaded with healthy fats, protein, and fiber, nuts and seeds like almonds, chia seeds, and flaxseeds support satiety, blood sugar control, and overall vitality.
- Turmeric: Contains curcumin, a powerful anti-inflammatory compound that may help reduce pain, improve joint health, and support immune function.
- Incorporating Superfoods into the Diet:
-
- Provide practical tips for incorporating superfoods into daily meals and snacks, such as adding berries to smoothies, salads, or oatmeal, incorporating leafy greens into soups, stir-fries, or salads, and sprinkling nuts and seeds on yogurt or salads.

- Offer creative recipe ideas that showcase the versatility and deliciousness of superfoods in a variety of cuisines and culinary styles.
- Synergy of Superfoods in a Balanced Diet:
-
- Discuss the concept of food synergy, which suggests that the combined effects of nutrients and phytochemicals in whole foods may be greater than the sum of their individual parts.
- Highlight the importance of consuming a diverse array of superfoods as part of a balanced diet to maximize their health benefits and support overall vitality.
- Cautionary Notes and Considerations:
-
- Acknowledge that while superfoods can provide valuable nutrients and health benefits, they are not a magic bullet for optimal health.
- Encourage moderation and variety in food choices, as excessive consumption of any single food may lead to nutrient imbalances or unwanted side effects.
- Conclusion: Harnessing the Power of Superfoods:
-
- Summarize the key benefits of superfoods and their potential to enhance vitality and well-being.
- Encourage readers to explore different superfoods, experiment with new recipes, and incorporate a variety of nutrient-rich foods into their diet to support lifelong health and vitality.
- Meal planning and portion control for optimal nutrition: How can we put all this knowledge into practice? We'll discuss strategies for meal planning, portion control, and mindful eating to ensure that we're nourishing our bodies with the right nutrients in the right amounts.

- Meal Planning and Portion Control for Optimal Nutrition
- Introduction to Meal Planning:
-
- Define meal planning as the process of organizing and preparing meals in advance to ensure they are balanced, nutritious, and aligned with personal health goals.
- Discuss the importance of meal planning for saving time, money, and energy, while also promoting healthier eating habits and better nutrition.
- Setting Health Goals and Priorities:
-
- Encourage readers to identify their health goals and priorities, such as weight management, improving energy levels, or supporting athletic performance.
- Discuss how understanding individual dietary preferences, food intolerances, and lifestyle factors can inform meal planning choices.
- Creating Balanced Meals:
-
- Provide guidelines for building balanced meals that include a variety of nutrient-rich foods from different food groups:
- Proteins: Include lean sources of protein such as poultry, fish, tofu, beans, or lentils.
- Carbohydrates: Choose complex carbohydrates like whole grains, fruits, and starchy vegetables.
- Vegetables: Aim to fill half of your plate with colorful vegetables for added vitamins, minerals, and fiber.
- Healthy Fats: Incorporate sources of healthy fats such as avocados, nuts, seeds, and olive oil.
- Portion Control: Discuss the importance of portion control in preventing overeating and promoting satiety. Offer practical tips for estimating portion

sizes using visual cues, measuring tools, or portion control containers.

- Meal Planning Strategies:

- Introduce different meal planning approaches and strategies to suit individual preferences and lifestyles, such as batch cooking, meal prepping, or using meal delivery services.
- Provide a step-by-step guide to meal planning, including:
- Menu Creation: Plan meals for the week ahead, considering factors like dietary preferences, nutritional balance, and available ingredients.
- Grocery Shopping: Compile a shopping list based on planned meals and ingredients needed to ensure you have everything on hand.
- Preparation: Set aside time for meal preparation, such as chopping vegetables, cooking proteins, or assembling ingredients for quick and easy meals during the week.
- Storage and Organization: Store prepared meals and ingredients properly to maintain freshness and minimize food waste.
- Smart Snacking and Hydration:

- Discuss the importance of incorporating healthy snacks and staying hydrated throughout the day to maintain energy levels and prevent overeating at mealtime.
- Offer suggestions for nutritious snacks that combine protein, carbohydrates, and healthy fats, such as Greek yogurt with fruit, veggies with hummus, or nuts and seeds.
- Emphasize the role of water in hydration and satiety, encouraging readers to drink water regularly

throughout the day and flavor it with fresh fruit or herbs for added variety.
- Flexibility and Adaptability:
-
- Encourage flexibility and adaptability in meal planning to accommodate changing schedules, unexpected events, or dining out occasions.
- Provide tips for making healthy choices when eating out or traveling, such as reviewing menus in advance, prioritizing vegetables and lean proteins, and practicing mindful eating habits.
- Tracking Progress and Adjusting as Needed:
-
- Suggest keeping a food diary or using a meal planning app to track meals, snacks, and overall dietary patterns.
- Encourage readers to reflect on their progress, identify areas for improvement, and make adjustments to their meal planning approach as needed to better align with their health goals and preferences.
- Conclusion: Empowering Nutritious Choices:
-
- Summarize the key principles of meal planning and portion control for optimal nutrition.
- Encourage readers to embrace meal planning as a tool for promoting healthier eating habits, supporting their health goals, and enjoying a balanced and nourishing diet.

Chapter 3: The Power of Movement

Now that we've covered the importance of nutrition, let's shift our focus to the role of physical activity in maintaining a healthy and vibrant life.

Chapter 3: The Power of Movement

Introduction to Physical Activity:

Define physical activity as any bodily movement produced by skeletal muscles that requires energy expenditure.

Discuss the importance of regular physical activity for overall health, well-being, and longevity.

Understanding the Benefits of Movement:

Explore the wide range of physical, mental, and emotional benefits associated with regular physical activity, including:

Physical Health: Improved cardiovascular health, enhanced muscular strength and endurance, better bone health, and reduced risk of chronic diseases such as obesity, type 2 diabetes, and certain cancers.

Mental Health: Reduced stress, anxiety, and depression symptoms, improved mood and self-esteem, and enhanced cognitive function and brain health.

Emotional Well-being: Increased energy levels, better sleep quality, and a greater sense of vitality and overall well-being.

Types of Physical Activity:

Discuss different types of physical activity and their respective benefits, including:

Aerobic Exercise: Activities that increase heart rate and breathing, such as walking, jogging, swimming, cycling, dancing, and aerobics.

Strength Training: Exercises that target muscle groups to build strength, endurance, and lean muscle mass, using body weight, free weights, resistance bands, or weight machines.

Flexibility and Balance Training: Activities that improve flexibility, mobility, and balance, such as yoga, Pilates, stretching, and tai chi.

Everyday Movement: Incorporating physical activity into daily routines through activities like gardening, housework, taking the stairs, or walking instead of driving.

Finding Your Movement Style:

Encourage readers to explore different types of physical activity and find activities they enjoy and can sustain long-term.

Offer tips for incorporating variety into workouts to prevent boredom, avoid plateaus, and challenge different muscle groups.

Overcoming Barriers to Physical Activity:

Identify common barriers to regular physical activity, such as lack of time, motivation, resources, or accessibility to fitness facilities.

Provide practical strategies for overcoming these barriers, such as setting realistic goals, scheduling workouts, enlisting social support, and finding creative ways to stay active.

Developing a Personalized Fitness Plan:

Guide readers through the process of creating a personalized fitness plan tailored to their individual goals, preferences, and fitness levels.

Discuss key components of a well-rounded fitness plan, including:

Frequency: How often to exercise (e.g., daily, several times a week).

Intensity: How hard to exercise, based on individual fitness levels and goals.

Duration: How long each workout session should last, depending on exercise intensity and type.

Progression: How to gradually increase exercise intensity, duration, or frequency over time to continue seeing improvements.

Incorporating Movement into Daily Life:

Offer practical tips for incorporating more movement into daily routines, such as:

Taking short activity breaks throughout the day (e.g., stretching, walking).

Parking farther away from destinations to increase walking distance.

Using active transportation options like biking or walking for errands or commuting.

Engaging in active hobbies and recreational activities that bring joy and fulfillment.

Staying Safe and Injury-Free:

Discuss the importance of proper form, technique, warm-up, and cool-down in preventing injuries during physical activity.

Offer guidance on listening to the body's cues, respecting physical limitations, and seeking professional guidance when needed.

Celebrating Progress and Staying Motivated:

Encourage readers to celebrate their achievements, no matter how small, and to focus on progress rather than perfection.

Provide strategies for staying motivated and overcoming obstacles, such as setting SMART goals, tracking progress, finding accountability partners, and rewarding oneself for reaching milestones.

Conclusion: Embracing the Power of Movement:

Summarize the key benefits of regular physical activity and its transformative impact on health and well-being.

Encourage readers to make movement a priority in their lives, embrace a more active lifestyle, and experience the profound benefits of regular physical activity firsthand.

- Finding an exercise routine that suits your lifestyle and goals: With so many exercise options available, how do we choose the right one for us? We'll explore different types of exercise, from strength training to yoga, and how to tailor our fitness routine to our individual needs and preferences.

- Incorporating strength training, cardio, and flexibility exercises into your regimen: What are the specific benefits of strength training, cardio, and flexibility exercises, and how can we incorporate them into our weekly routine? We'll discuss the unique advantages of each type of exercise and how they work together to support our overall fitness.
- Overcoming barriers to physical activity and staying motivated: Many of us struggle to maintain a consistent exercise routine. How can we overcome common barriers like lack of time, motivation, or confidence? We'll share practical tips for staying motivated and committed to regular physical activity.

Chapter 4: Rest and Recovery

In this chapter, we'll explore the often overlooked but crucial aspects of rest and recovery for overall health and vitality.

Chapter 4: Rest and Recovery

Introduction to Rest and Recovery:

Define rest and recovery as essential components of any well-rounded fitness and wellness regimen.

Discuss the importance of rest and recovery for optimizing performance, preventing injury, and promoting overall health and well-being.

Understanding the Restorative Power of Sleep:

Explore the vital role of sleep in physical, mental, and emotional restoration and repair.

Discuss the stages of sleep, including deep sleep and REM sleep, and their respective functions in memory consolidation, hormone regulation, and immune function.

The Benefits of Adequate Sleep:

Highlight the numerous health benefits associated with getting sufficient, high-quality sleep, including:

Physical Health: Improved immune function, reduced inflammation, better cardiovascular health, and lower risk of obesity and chronic diseases.

Mental Health: Enhanced cognitive function, better mood regulation, and reduced risk of anxiety and depression.

Athletic Performance: Improved reaction time, coordination, and muscle recovery, leading to better athletic performance and injury prevention.

Establishing Healthy Sleep Habits:

Provide practical tips for improving sleep quality and duration, such as:

Maintaining a consistent sleep schedule by going to bed and waking up at the same time each day.

Creating a relaxing bedtime routine to signal the body that it's time to wind down (e.g., dimming lights, practicing relaxation techniques).

Creating a sleep-friendly environment by keeping the bedroom cool, dark, and quiet, and removing electronic devices that emit blue light.

The Importance of Active Recovery:

Discuss the concept of active recovery as a deliberate strategy to facilitate muscle repair, reduce soreness, and promote faster recovery after intense exercise.

Explore different forms of active recovery, such as low-intensity exercise, yoga, stretching, foam rolling, and massage therapy.

Nutrition and Hydration for Recovery:

Highlight the role of nutrition and hydration in supporting post-exercise recovery and replenishing glycogen stores, repairing muscle tissue, and reducing inflammation.

Provide guidelines for post-workout nutrition, including consuming a combination of carbohydrates and protein within the first hour after exercise to optimize recovery.

Mindful Rest and Stress Management:

Discuss the importance of incorporating periods of rest and relaxation into daily routines to manage stress levels and prevent burnout.

Offer strategies for practicing mindfulness, meditation, deep breathing exercises, and other stress-reducing techniques to promote relaxation and mental well-being.

The Art of Balancing Activity and Rest:

Emphasize the importance of finding a balance between physical activity and restorative rest to avoid overtraining, fatigue, and injury.

Discuss the signs of overtraining and the importance of listening to the body's signals to prevent pushing beyond its limits.

Sleep Disorders and Seeking Professional Help:

Acknowledge the prevalence of sleep disorders such as insomnia, sleep apnea, and restless leg syndrome, and their impact on overall health and quality of life.

Encourage readers to seek professional help if they experience persistent sleep disturbances or suspect they may have a sleep disorder that requires diagnosis and treatment.

Conclusion: Embracing Rest and Recovery:

Summarize the key principles of rest and recovery and their importance for optimizing health, performance, and overall well-being.

Encourage readers to prioritize restorative rest and recovery practices as essential components of their fitness and wellness journey, and to reap the benefits of a balanced approach to physical activity and relaxation.

- The importance of quality sleep and its impact on cognitive function and physical health: What exactly happens when we sleep, and why is it so important for our well-being? We'll delve into the science of sleep and its profound effects on cognition, mood, immune function, and more.
- Strategies for improving sleep hygiene and establishing a bedtime routine: How can we improve the quality of our sleep and establish healthy bedtime habits? We'll discuss practical strategies for creating a soothing sleep environment and developing a relaxing pre-sleep routine.
- Techniques for managing stress and promoting relaxation: Stress can take a toll on our physical and mental health. What are some effective techniques for managing stress and promoting relaxation, even in the midst of a busy and demanding lifestyle? We'll explore mindfulness, meditation, and other stress-reducing practices.

Chapter 5: Mental and Emotional Well-being

Introduction to Mental and Emotional Well-being:

Define mental and emotional well-being as the state of overall psychological health, encompassing feelings of happiness, fulfillment, and resilience in the face of life's challenges.

Discuss the interconnectedness of mental and emotional health with physical health and overall quality of life.

Understanding Mental Health:

Define mental health and explore common mental health disorders, such as anxiety disorders, mood disorders (e.g., depression, bipolar disorder), and psychotic disorders.

Discuss the prevalence of mental health conditions and the importance of destigmatizing mental illness.

Promoting Emotional Resilience:

Discuss the concept of emotional resilience as the ability to bounce back from adversity, cope with stress, and adapt to change.

Offer strategies for building emotional resilience, such as cultivating a positive mindset, practicing self-compassion, and developing healthy coping mechanisms.

Stress Management Techniques:

Explore various stress management techniques and relaxation strategies to promote mental and emotional well-being, including:

Mindfulness and Meditation: Practices that involve focusing attention on the present moment, cultivating awareness, and reducing reactivity to stressors.

Deep Breathing Exercises: Techniques that promote relaxation by slowing down the breath and activating the body's relaxation response.

Progressive Muscle Relaxation: Exercises that involve tensing and relaxing muscle groups to release physical tension and promote relaxation.

Yoga and Tai Chi: Mind-body practices that combine physical movement with breath awareness and meditation to reduce stress and improve mental clarity.

Nurturing Positive Relationships:

Highlight the importance of social connections and supportive relationships for mental and emotional well-being.

Offer tips for building and maintaining positive relationships, such as effective communication, active listening, empathy, and conflict resolution skills.

Practicing Gratitude and Mindfulness:

Discuss the benefits of practicing gratitude and mindfulness for promoting mental and emotional well-being, including increased happiness, resilience, and overall life satisfaction.

Provide practical exercises and techniques for incorporating gratitude and mindfulness into daily routines, such as keeping a gratitude journal, practicing mindful breathing, or engaging in daily acts of kindness.

Seeking Professional Help and Support:

Acknowledge that seeking professional help is a sign of strength and courage, not weakness.

Provide information on accessing mental health services, including therapy, counseling, support groups, and hotlines, for individuals experiencing mental health challenges.

Self-care Practices for Mental Health:

Discuss the importance of self-care practices for nurturing mental and emotional well-being, such as:

Physical Activity: Regular exercise to boost mood, reduce stress, and improve overall mental health.

Healthy Lifestyle Habits: Prioritizing sleep, nutrition, hydration, and relaxation to support mental and emotional resilience.

Creative Expression: Engaging in creative activities such as art, music, writing, or gardening as outlets for self-expression and emotional release.

Cultivating Meaning and Purpose:

Explore the importance of finding meaning and purpose in life for promoting mental and emotional well-being.

Offer guidance on identifying personal values, goals, and passions, and incorporating them into daily life to foster a sense of fulfillment and satisfaction.

Conclusion: Embracing Mental and Emotional Well-being:

Summarize the key principles of promoting mental and emotional well-being and their significance for overall health and quality of life.

Encourage readers to prioritize self-care, seek support when needed, and cultivate resilience, gratitude, and positive relationships to thrive in all aspects of life.

Our mental and emotional well-being is just as important as our physical health. In this chapter, we'll explore the crucial

role of our mindset and emotions in achieving overall
vitality.

- Understanding the mind-body connection and its
  influence on overall health: How does our mental
  and emotional state impact our physical health, and
  vice versa? We'll discuss the powerful connection
  between our thoughts, emotions, and bodily
  functions, and how we can harness this connection
  for our well-being.
- Techniques for managing stress, anxiety, and
  negative emotions: Everyone experiences stress and
  negative emotions from time to time. What are
  some practical techniques for managing these
  feelings and cultivating a more positive mindset?
  We'll explore tools such as cognitive reframing,
  journaling, and gratitude practices.
- Cultivating mindfulness and gratitude for a positive
  outlook on life: Mindfulness and gratitude have
  been shown to have profound effects on overall
  well-being. How can we integrate these practices
  into our daily lives to foster a more positive and
  resilient mindset? We'll share simple yet powerful
  exercises for cultivating mindfulness and gratitude.

Chapter 6: Building Healthy Habits

Now that we've covered the foundational principles of health and well-being, let's shift our focus to the practical aspects of building and sustaining healthy habits.

Chapter 6: Building Healthy Habits

Introduction to Healthy Habits:

Define healthy habits as behaviors that contribute to overall well-being and support long-term health and vitality.

Discuss the importance of building and maintaining healthy habits for achieving health goals and sustaining lifestyle changes.

Understanding Habit Formation:

Explore the science of habit formation and behavior change, including the habit loop (cue, routine, reward) and the concept of habit stacking.

Discuss factors that influence habit formation, such as motivation, consistency, environment, and social support.

Identifying Core Health Habits:

Introduce key health habits that form the foundation of a healthy lifestyle, including:

Nutrition: Making balanced, nutritious food choices and practicing mindful eating habits.

Physical Activity: Incorporating regular exercise and movement into daily routines to support physical fitness and overall well-being.

Sleep: Prioritizing sufficient, high-quality sleep to promote physical and mental health.

Stress Management: Implementing stress-reducing techniques and relaxation practices to support mental and emotional resilience.

Hydration: Maintaining adequate hydration levels by drinking plenty of water throughout the day.

Self-care: Nurturing mental, emotional, and physical well-being through self-care practices such as mindfulness, relaxation, and leisure activities.

Setting SMART Goals:

Discuss the importance of setting specific, measurable, achievable, relevant, and time-bound (SMART) goals for building and sustaining healthy habits.

Provide guidance on setting SMART goals for different areas of health and well-being, such as nutrition, fitness, sleep, and stress management.

Creating a Healthy Habit Action Plan:

Offer a step-by-step process for creating a personalized action plan for building and reinforcing healthy habits, including:

Identifying Target Habits: Choosing one or two specific habits to focus on initially, based on individual goals and priorities.

Breaking Down Goals: Breaking larger goals into smaller, manageable action steps to increase likelihood of success.

Implementing Behavior Change Strategies: Using techniques such as habit stacking, positive reinforcement, and environmental cues to support habit formation.

Tracking Progress: Monitoring and evaluating progress regularly to identify successes and areas for improvement.

Overcoming Common Challenges:

Address common challenges and obstacles to building and maintaining healthy habits, such as lack of motivation, time constraints, stress, or social pressures.

Provide practical strategies for overcoming these challenges, such as:

Creating Accountability: Enlisting support from friends, family members, or accountability partners to stay motivated and accountable.

Managing Setbacks: Developing resilience and coping strategies to bounce back from setbacks and continue making progress toward health goals.

Adjusting Goals as Needed: Being flexible and willing to adjust goals and action plans based on changing circumstances or feedback.

Celebrating Success and Staying Motivated:

Emphasize the importance of celebrating successes, no matter how small, and acknowledging progress along the journey.

Offer tips for staying motivated and maintaining momentum, such as rewarding oneself for achieving milestones, visualizing success, and cultivating a growth mindset.

Creating a Supportive Environment:

Discuss the role of environment in shaping behavior and habits, and offer strategies for creating a supportive environment conducive to healthy living.

Provide tips for organizing living spaces, stocking pantries with nutritious foods, and surrounding oneself with supportive social networks.

Lifelong Learning and Adaptability:

Encourage a mindset of lifelong learning and growth, embracing opportunities to learn from successes and setbacks alike.

Discuss the importance of adaptability and flexibility in adjusting habits and behaviors as circumstances change over time.

Conclusion: Cultivating Lasting Change:

Summarize the key principles of building healthy habits and their transformative impact on health and well-being.

Encourage readers to commit to their health goals, embrace the process of habit formation, and take proactive steps to cultivate a lifestyle that supports long-term health, vitality, and fulfillment.

- The science of habit formation and how to create lasting change: How do habits form, and how can we leverage this knowledge to create lasting changes in our behavior? We'll explore the science of habit formation and practical strategies for establishing new, healthy habits.
- Strategies for breaking bad habits and replacing them with positive behaviors: Many of us struggle

with breaking unhealthy habits. What are some
effective strategies for letting go of detrimental
behaviors and replacing them with healthier
alternatives? We'll discuss the process of habit
replacement and how to navigate common
obstacles.
- Setting realistic goals and tracking progress for
  long-term success: Goal-setting and progress
  tracking are essential for maintaining motivation
  and momentum on our wellness journey. How can
  we set realistic, achievable goals and measure our
  progress effectively? We'll share tips for setting
  meaningful goals and tracking our success along the
  way.

Chapter 7: The Role of Relationships

Our relationships and social connections have a profound impact on our overall well-being. In this chapter, we'll explore the importance of nurturing healthy relationships for vitality.

Introduction to Relationships:

Define relationships as connections between individuals characterized by mutual respect, trust, and support.

Discuss the importance of relationships for overall well-being and quality of life.

Types of Relationships:

Explore different types of relationships that contribute to social connectedness and support, including:

Family Relationships: Bonds with parents, siblings, children, and extended family members.

Friendships: Connections with peers and acquaintances based on shared interests, values, and experiences.

Romantic Relationships: Intimate partnerships characterized by love, commitment, and mutual affection.

Professional Relationships: Interactions with colleagues, mentors, supervisors, and clients in work or academic settings.

Community Connections: Involvement in social groups, clubs, or organizations within the local community.

The Impact of Relationships on Health and Well-being:

Discuss the profound influence of relationships on physical, mental, and emotional health, including:

Social Support: The role of supportive relationships in buffering against stress, reducing risk of depression, and promoting resilience.

Emotional Intimacy: The importance of emotional connection and communication in fostering feelings of belonging, security, and fulfillment.

Health Behaviors: How relationships can influence health behaviors such as exercise, nutrition, and substance use through social norms, modeling, and support.

Longevity: Research on the association between strong social ties and increased longevity and overall well-being.

Building Healthy Relationships:

Provide guidance on cultivating healthy relationships characterized by trust, communication, and mutual respect, including:

Effective Communication: Active listening, assertiveness, and empathy as key components of healthy communication.

Boundaries: Establishing and respecting personal boundaries to maintain autonomy and self-respect within relationships.

Conflict Resolution: Strategies for resolving conflicts constructively, such as compromise, negotiation, and seeking common ground.

Supportive Dynamics: Nurturing supportive dynamics within relationships through empathy, validation, and encouragement.

Navigating Challenging Relationships:

Acknowledge that not all relationships are positive or healthy, and provide guidance on navigating challenging relationships, including:

Setting Limits: Establishing boundaries and limits in toxic or abusive relationships to protect one's well-being.

Seeking Support: Reaching out to trusted friends, family members, or professionals for guidance and support in navigating difficult relationships.

Self-Care: Prioritizing self-care practices to maintain emotional resilience and protect against the negative impact of challenging relationships.

Cultivating Connection in the Digital Age:

Discuss the impact of technology and social media on interpersonal relationships, and offer strategies for cultivating meaningful connections in the digital age, such as:

Balancing Screen Time: Setting boundaries around device use to prioritize face-to-face interactions and quality time with loved ones.

Authentic Communication: Fostering authentic connections through genuine interactions and vulnerability, both online and offline.

Mindful Engagement: Practicing mindfulness and presence in online interactions to foster deeper connections and reduce the risk of social comparison and loneliness.

Nurturing Romantic Relationships:

Offer guidance on nurturing healthy, fulfilling romantic relationships characterized by trust, intimacy, and mutual respect, including:

Communication and Connection: Prioritizing open and honest communication, emotional intimacy, and quality time together.

Shared Values and Goals: Aligning values, goals, and priorities to foster a sense of partnership and mutual support.

Conflict Resolution: Approaching conflicts with empathy, respect, and a willingness to work through differences constructively.

Supporting Friendships and Social Connections:

Discuss the importance of friendships and social connections for overall well-being, and offer tips for nurturing and maintaining meaningful friendships, such as:

Quality Time: Making time for regular social interactions and meaningful conversations with friends.

Reciprocity: Fostering mutual support, reciprocity, and shared activities within friendships.

Diverse Social Networks: Cultivating diverse social networks and exploring new interests and hobbies to expand social circles and opportunities for connection.

Fostering Family Bonds:

Explore the unique dynamics of family relationships and offer strategies for fostering strong, supportive family bonds, such as:

Communication and Understanding: Cultivating open communication, empathy, and understanding within family relationships.

Quality Time: Prioritizing regular family rituals, traditions, and shared experiences to strengthen family bonds.

Conflict Resolution: Approaching conflicts with patience, compassion, and a commitment to finding mutually acceptable solutions.

Conclusion: Embracing Connection and Support:

Summarize the importance of relationships for overall health, happiness, and well-being.

Encourage readers to prioritize building and nurturing meaningful relationships, invest in their social connections, and seek support and connection to thrive in all aspects of life.

Introduction to Relationships:

Relationships are the connections we have with others, forming the fabric of our social lives. They can include family, friends, romantic partners, colleagues, and community members. Relationships contribute significantly to our sense of belonging, identity, and overall well-being.

Types of Relationships:

There are various types of relationships, each serving different purposes and providing unique forms of support and companionship. Family relationships are often the most foundational, providing a sense of identity and belonging.

Friendships offer companionship, shared experiences, and emotional support. Romantic relationships provide intimacy, love, and partnership. Professional relationships support career development and collaboration, while community connections foster a sense of belonging and civic engagement.

The Impact of Relationships on Health and Well-being:

Strong, supportive relationships have a profound impact on our health and well-being. They provide emotional support during challenging times, reduce stress, and promote resilience. Healthy relationships can positively influence health behaviors, such as encouraging regular exercise or providing a supportive environment for healthy eating habits. Research also suggests that strong social ties are associated with increased longevity and overall life satisfaction.

Building Healthy Relationships:

Healthy relationships are built on a foundation of mutual respect, trust, and effective communication. Effective communication involves active listening, expressing thoughts and feelings honestly and respectfully, and being open to feedback. Setting boundaries is also crucial for maintaining healthy relationships, as it establishes expectations and protects individual autonomy and well-being. Conflict resolution skills are essential for addressing disagreements constructively and preserving relationship harmony.

Navigating Challenging Relationships:

Not all relationships are positive or healthy, and navigating challenging relationships can be difficult. Setting limits and boundaries is essential for protecting one's well-being in toxic or abusive relationships. Seeking support from trusted individuals or professionals can provide guidance and validation during challenging times. Practicing self-care and prioritizing emotional resilience are crucial for maintaining well-being in the face of difficult relationships.

Cultivating Connection in the Digital Age:

In today's digital age, technology and social media play a significant role in how we connect with others. While technology can facilitate communication and connection, it's essential to balance screen time with face-to-face interactions and prioritize meaningful connections. Authentic communication and mindful engagement in online interactions can help foster deeper connections and reduce feelings of loneliness and social isolation.

Nurturing Romantic Relationships:

Romantic relationships require intentional effort to maintain intimacy, trust, and connection. Effective communication, emotional intimacy, and shared values and goals are essential for nurturing healthy, fulfilling partnerships. Conflict resolution skills and a willingness to work through differences constructively are also vital for preserving relationship harmony and mutual understanding.

Supporting Friendships and Social Connections:

Friendships and social connections are vital for our mental and emotional well-being. Nurturing friendships involves making time for quality interactions, fostering reciprocity and shared activities, and cultivating diverse social networks. Building and maintaining friendships require effort and investment but can provide significant rewards in terms of companionship, support, and shared experiences.

Fostering Family Bonds:

Family relationships are among the most significant and enduring connections in our lives. Fostering strong family bonds involves effective communication, quality time spent together, and resolving conflicts with patience and understanding. Family rituals, traditions, and shared experiences help strengthen family connections and create lasting memories.

Conclusion: Embracing Connection and Support:

Relationships are essential for our overall health, happiness, and well-being. Prioritizing meaningful connections, investing in social support networks, and seeking support when needed are crucial for thriving in all aspects of life. Embracing connection and support enriches our lives and contributes to our sense of fulfillment and belonging.

- The impact of social connections on mental and physical health: How do our relationships and social connections influence our mental and physical well-being? We'll delve into the research on the health benefits of strong social ties and the detrimental effects of social isolation.
- Nurturing healthy relationships and setting boundaries for self-care: What does it mean to nurture healthy relationships, and how can we establish boundaries to protect our well-being? We'll discuss the importance of healthy communication, mutual support, and self-care within our relationships.
- Strategies for managing conflict and fostering a supportive network: Conflict is a natural part of any relationship. What are some effective strategies for managing conflict constructively and fostering a supportive network of friends, family, and colleagues? We'll explore techniques for effective communication, conflict resolution, and building a strong support system.

Chapter 8: Creating a Healthy Environment

Our physical surroundings play a significant role in our overall well-being. In this chapter, we'll explore the impact of our environment on our health and vitality.

Environmental health refers to the interactions between human health and the surrounding environment, encompassing physical, chemical, biological, and social factors that influence health outcomes.

This chapter explores how individuals can create and maintain healthy environments in their homes, workplaces, communities, and broader surroundings to support overall well-being.

Understanding Environmental Influences on Health:

Discuss the various ways in which environmental factors impact human health, including:

Physical Environment: The quality of air, water, and soil, as well as exposure to natural disasters and hazards, can affect respiratory health, waterborne illnesses, and injuries.

Chemical Exposures: Exposure to pollutants, toxins, and hazardous substances in the environment can lead to adverse health effects, such as respiratory problems, neurological disorders, and cancer.

Biological Agents: Infectious agents, allergens, and vector-borne diseases transmitted by insects or animals can pose health risks in certain environments.

Social and Built Environment: Social determinants of health, such as socioeconomic status, access to healthcare, and community infrastructure, also influence health outcomes and disparities.

Creating a Healthy Home Environment:

Offer guidance on creating a healthy home environment by:

Improving Indoor Air Quality: Ventilating indoor spaces, minimizing indoor pollutants (e.g., tobacco smoke, volatile organic compounds), and using air purifiers to reduce allergens and contaminants.

Ensuring Safe Drinking Water: Testing drinking water quality regularly, using water filters if necessary, and avoiding exposure to lead, arsenic, and other contaminants in drinking water.

Promoting Safety: Implementing safety measures to prevent accidents and injuries, such as installing smoke alarms, carbon monoxide detectors, and childproofing measures.

Reducing Exposure to Toxins: Minimizing exposure to household chemicals, pesticides, and other toxic substances by choosing natural cleaning products, organic foods, and non-toxic household materials.

Creating a Healthy Work Environment:

Discuss strategies for promoting health and well-being in the workplace by:

Encouraging Physical Activity: Providing opportunities for physical activity breaks, ergonomic workstations, and active commuting options (e.g., walking or biking to work).

Supporting Mental Health: Offering resources and programs to support employee mental health and well-being, such as stress management workshops, employee assistance programs, and flexible work arrangements.

Promoting Work-Life Balance: Encouraging work-life balance through flexible schedules, telecommuting options, and policies that support parental leave and caregiving responsibilities.

Ensuring Occupational Safety: Implementing safety protocols, training programs, and ergonomic practices to prevent workplace injuries and illnesses.

Creating Healthy Community Environments:

Explore ways to promote health and well-being at the community level by:

Supporting Access to Healthy Foods: Increasing access to fresh, nutritious foods through farmers' markets, community gardens, and food assistance programs in underserved areas.

Creating Active Living Spaces: Designing walkable neighborhoods, bike lanes, parks, and recreational facilities to encourage physical activity and social interaction.

Addressing Environmental Justice: Advocating for equitable access to clean air, safe drinking water, and healthy living conditions for all community members, particularly marginalized and vulnerable populations.

Building Social Connections: Fostering social cohesion, community engagement, and civic participation through neighborhood associations, community events, and volunteer opportunities.

Promoting Sustainable Practices:

Emphasize the importance of adopting sustainable practices to protect the environment and human health by:

Reducing Waste: Minimizing waste generation through recycling, composting, and reducing single-use plastics and packaging.

Conserving Resources: Conserving energy and water resources through energy-efficient appliances, renewable energy sources, and water-saving technologies.

Protecting Natural Habitats: Preserving and restoring natural habitats, biodiversity, and green spaces to support ecosystem health and resilience.

Advocating for Policy Change: Engaging in advocacy efforts to promote environmental policies and regulations that protect public health and the planet, such as climate action initiatives, pollution control measures, and sustainable urban planning.

Creating Supportive Social Environments:

Highlight the importance of creating supportive social environments that foster belonging, connection, and social support by:

Building Social Networks: Cultivating meaningful relationships, participating in community activities, and seeking out social support networks in times of need.

Promoting Inclusivity and Diversity: Creating inclusive spaces that embrace diversity, equity, and inclusion and celebrate cultural differences and perspectives.

Addressing Social Determinants of Health: Advocating for policies and programs that address social determinants of health, such as affordable housing, education, employment opportunities, and healthcare access.

Conclusion: Empowering Environmental Health:

Summarize the key principles of creating and maintaining healthy environments to support human health and well-being.

Encourage readers to take proactive steps to promote environmental health in their homes, workplaces, communities, and broader

Physical Environment:

Our physical environment includes elements such as air quality, water quality, natural landscapes, buildings, and infrastructure. These factors can directly influence our well-being in several ways:

Air Quality: Poor air quality, due to pollution or allergens, can exacerbate respiratory conditions like asthma and allergies, leading to discomfort and health complications.

Water Quality: Contaminated water sources can pose health risks, including gastrointestinal illnesses and exposure to harmful chemicals or pathogens.

Natural Landscapes: Access to green spaces, parks, and natural landscapes has been linked to reduced stress, improved mood, and enhanced cognitive function.

Built Environment: Well-designed buildings and urban spaces can promote physical activity, social interaction, and community cohesion, contributing to overall well-being.

Social Environment:

Our social environment encompasses interactions with family, friends, peers, colleagues, and the broader community. Social connections and support networks profoundly influence our well-being:

Social Support: Strong social connections provide emotional support, companionship, and a sense of belonging, buffering against stress and promoting resilience.

Social Norms and Expectations: Social norms and cultural expectations within our social environment shape behaviors, attitudes, and perceptions of health and well-being.

Stress and Social Isolation: Social stressors, such as conflicts or social isolation, can negatively impact mental health, increasing the risk of depression, anxiety, and other psychological disorders.

Community Resources and Services: Access to community resources, such as healthcare facilities, social services, and recreational amenities, plays a vital role in promoting well-being and quality of life.

Psychological Environment:

Our psychological environment encompasses internal factors such as thoughts, beliefs, attitudes, and perceptions, which are influenced by external surroundings:

Perceived Safety and Security: Feelings of safety and security within our environment contribute to a sense of well-being and peace of mind.

Psychological Comfort: Environments that are aesthetically pleasing, organized, and conducive to relaxation promote psychological comfort and emotional well-being.

Stress and Environmental Stimuli: Environmental stimuli, such as noise, crowding, or clutter, can trigger stress responses and negatively impact mental health and cognitive function.

Cultural and Social Context: Cultural values, beliefs, and social norms shape our perceptions of well-being and influence behaviors related to health, relationships, and lifestyle choices.

Overall, understanding the influence of our surroundings on our well-being involves recognizing the interconnectedness of physical, social, and psychological factors in shaping our health outcomes and quality of life. By creating environments that promote safety, social connection, and psychological comfort, we can enhance our overall well-being and resilience in the face of life's challenges.

- Understanding the influence of our surroundings on our well-being: How does our physical environment, including our home, workplace, and community, impact our health and vitality? We'll examine the ways in which our surroundings can either support or detract from our well-being.
- Tips for decluttering and organizing your space for mental clarity: A cluttered and disorganized environment can contribute to stress and overwhelm. What are some practical tips for decluttering and organizing our living and working spaces to promote mental clarity and a sense of calm? We'll discuss strategies for creating an environment that supports our well-being.
- Incorporating nature and natural elements into daily life for a sense of calm and balance: Nature has a powerful impact on our mental and emotional well-being. How can we incorporate natural elements into our daily lives, even in urban environments, to

promote a sense of calm and balance? We'll explore simple ways to connect with nature and reap its rejuvenating benefits.

Chapter 9: Preventative Health Measures

Preventative Health Measures

Introduction to Preventative Health:

Preventative health measures are proactive strategies aimed at reducing the risk of illness, injury, and chronic diseases before they occur. This chapter explores various preventative measures individuals can take to promote their health and well-being.

Importance of Preventative Health:

Discuss the significance of preventative health in reducing healthcare costs, improving quality of life, and extending lifespan. Emphasize that prevention is often more effective and less costly than treatment, making it a critical component of healthcare.

Physical Activity and Exercise:

Highlight the role of regular physical activity and exercise in preventing chronic diseases such as obesity, diabetes, heart disease, and certain types of cancer. Discuss recommendations for aerobic exercise, strength training, and flexibility exercises, and provide tips for incorporating physical activity into daily routines.

Healthy Eating Habits:

Discuss the importance of a balanced diet rich in fruits, vegetables, whole grains, lean proteins, and healthy fats for preventing chronic diseases and maintaining optimal health. Offer practical tips for making healthier food choices, meal planning, and portion control.

Regular Health Screenings:

Emphasize the importance of regular health screenings for early detection and prevention of common health conditions, such as hypertension, high cholesterol, diabetes, and certain cancers. Provide recommendations for age-appropriate screenings and preventive healthcare visits.

Immunizations and Vaccinations:

Discuss the role of immunizations and vaccinations in preventing infectious diseases and protecting public health. Highlight the importance of staying up-to-date on recommended vaccinations for children, adolescents, and adults to prevent outbreaks and reduce the spread of vaccine-preventable diseases.

Maintaining a Healthy Weight:

Explore the health risks associated with obesity and overweight, including an increased risk of heart disease, stroke, type 2 diabetes, and certain cancers. Offer strategies for achieving and maintaining a healthy weight through a combination of healthy eating, regular physical activity, and behavioral changes.

Stress Management and Relaxation Techniques:

Discuss the impact of chronic stress on health and well-being, including increased risk of cardiovascular disease, depression, anxiety, and other health problems. Provide evidence-based stress management techniques, such as mindfulness meditation, deep breathing exercises, progressive muscle relaxation, and yoga, to promote relaxation and reduce stress.

Healthy Sleep Habits:

Highlight the importance of adequate sleep for overall health and well-being, including cognitive function, mood regulation, immune function, and cardiovascular health. Offer tips for improving sleep hygiene, such as maintaining a consistent sleep schedule, creating a relaxing bedtime routine, and creating a sleep-friendly environment.

Avoiding Tobacco, Alcohol, and Substance Abuse:

Discuss the health risks associated with tobacco use, excessive alcohol consumption, and substance abuse, including increased risk of cancer, liver disease, addiction, and mental health disorders. Provide strategies for tobacco cessation, moderation of alcohol consumption, and seeking help for substance abuse.

Sun Protection and Skin Health:

Educate readers on the importance of sun protection for preventing skin cancer and premature aging. Offer recommendations for using sunscreen, wearing protective clothing, seeking shade, and avoiding indoor tanning beds to reduce sun exposure and protect skin health.

Injury Prevention and Safety Measures:

Discuss common types of injuries and accidents, such as falls, motor vehicle accidents, burns, and poisoning, and offer strategies for preventing injuries and promoting safety at home, work, and in recreational activities. Provide guidance on using safety equipment, practicing safe behaviors, and recognizing potential hazards.

Maintaining Mental and Emotional Health:

Explore the connection between mental and emotional health and overall well-being. Offer strategies for promoting mental and emotional resilience, such as stress management techniques, social support, self-care practices, and seeking professional help when needed.

Conclusion: Empowering Prevention:

Summarize the key preventative health measures discussed in the chapter and emphasize the importance of taking proactive steps to safeguard health and well-being. Encourage readers to prioritize prevention as a fundamental aspect of self-care and to take ownership of their health through healthy lifestyle choices and preventative healthcare practices.

In this chapter, we'll explore the importance of proactive health measures for preventing illness and maintaining vitality.

- The importance of regular check-ups and screenings for early detection of health issues: Regular preventive care and screenings are essential for catching potential health issues early. How can we prioritize and stay on top of these crucial check-ups and tests? We'll discuss the importance of preventive care and strategies for staying proactive about our health.
- Understanding the role of vaccines, immunizations, and preventive care: Vaccines and immunizations are vital tools for preventing infectious diseases. How do these preventive measures work, and why are they important for our overall health and well-being? We'll explore the science behind vaccines

and the benefits of staying up to date with immunizations.
- Incorporating holistic and alternative health practices for comprehensive well-being: In addition to conventional medical care, holistic and alternative health practices can play a valuable role in maintaining overall well-being. What are some examples of these practices, and how can we integrate them into our wellness routine? We'll discuss approaches such as acupuncture, herbal medicine, and mind-body therapies.

Chapter 10: The Journey to Lifelong Vitality

As we near the end of our journey through the secrets of a healthy life, let's explore how we can maintain vitality and well-being throughout our lives.

Lifelong vitality refers to the pursuit of optimal health, energy, and well-being throughout every stage of life. This chapter explores the multifaceted journey towards achieving and maintaining vitality, encompassing physical, mental, emotional, and spiritual aspects of health.

Understanding Vitality:

Define vitality as the state of being full of life, energy, and vigor. Discuss the components of vitality, including physical health, mental clarity, emotional resilience, and spiritual fulfillment. Emphasize that vitality is not just about longevity but about thriving and living life to the fullest.

Holistic Approach to Health:

Advocate for a holistic approach to health that addresses the interconnectedness of mind, body, and spirit. Highlight the importance of balancing physical, mental, emotional, and spiritual well-being to achieve optimal vitality and overall health.

Nutrition for Vitality:

Discuss the role of nutrition in supporting vitality and longevity. Emphasize the importance of a balanced diet rich in fruits, vegetables, whole grains, lean proteins, and healthy fats for providing essential nutrients, antioxidants, and phytochemicals that promote health and vitality. Provide guidance on making nutritious food choices, meal planning, and portion control to support vitality.

Physical Activity and Exercise:

Highlight the benefits of regular physical activity and exercise for promoting vitality and longevity. Discuss the role of exercise in improving cardiovascular health, strength, flexibility, and overall fitness. Encourage a variety of physical activities, including aerobic exercise, strength training, flexibility exercises, and mind-body practices such as yoga and tai chi, to support vitality and well-being.

Stress Management and Resilience:

Explore strategies for managing stress and cultivating resilience to promote vitality and overall well-being. Provide evidence-based stress management techniques, such as mindfulness meditation, deep breathing exercises, progressive muscle relaxation, and cognitive-behavioral strategies, to reduce stress and enhance coping skills. Discuss the importance of self-care practices, social support, and healthy lifestyle habits in building resilience and maintaining vitality.

Emotional Well-being and Connection:

Discuss the importance of emotional well-being and meaningful connections in promoting vitality and life satisfaction. Explore strategies for nurturing positive relationships, fostering emotional intimacy, and cultivating a sense of belonging and purpose. Highlight the role of empathy, compassion, and gratitude in enhancing emotional well-being and fostering resilience.

Mindfulness and Presence:

Advocate for mindfulness and presence as essential practices for enhancing vitality and living in the present moment. Discuss the benefits of mindfulness meditation, mindful eating, and mindful movement in promoting relaxation, stress reduction, and emotional balance. Provide practical tips for incorporating mindfulness into daily life and cultivating a greater sense of awareness and appreciation for the present moment.

Meaning and Purpose:

Explore the importance of finding meaning and purpose in life as a key component of vitality and well-being. Discuss the connection between a sense of purpose, personal fulfillment, and overall life satisfaction. Encourage readers to explore their values, passions, and goals to cultivate a sense of meaning and direction in their lives.

Self-Reflection and Growth:

Advocate for self-reflection and personal growth as ongoing processes in the journey to lifelong vitality. Discuss the benefits of self-awareness, self-discovery, and continuous learning in promoting personal development and fulfillment. Encourage readers to embrace challenges, setbacks, and opportunities for growth as integral parts of the journey to vitality.

Cultivating Gratitude and Joy:

Highlight the importance of cultivating gratitude and joy as practices for enhancing vitality and well-being. Discuss the benefits of gratitude practices, such as keeping a gratitude journal, expressing appreciation, and savoring positive experiences. Encourage readers to focus on the present moment, find joy in simple pleasures, and cultivate an attitude of gratitude in their daily lives.

Conclusion: Embracing the Journey:

Summarize the key principles of the journey to lifelong vitality, including nutrition, physical activity, stress management, emotional well-being, mindfulness, meaning, and personal growth. Encourage readers to embrace the journey to vitality as a lifelong pursuit, filled with opportunities for self-discovery, growth, and fulfillment. Encourage readers to prioritize self-care, cultivate resilience, and live with purpose and intention to maximize their vitality and well-being throughout every stage of life.

- Embracing the concept of aging with grace and vitality: Aging is a natural part of life, but it doesn't have to mean a decline in vitality. How can we embrace the process of aging with grace and maintain our well-being as we grow older? We'll explore the positive aspects of aging and strategies for staying vibrant at every stage of life.
- Strategies for maintaining healthy habits as life circumstances change: Life is full of changes, and our wellness journey will inevitably evolve along with our circumstances. How can we adapt and maintain healthy habits through life transitions, such as career changes, parenthood, or retirement? We'll discuss strategies for flexibility and resilience in the face of change.
- Cultivating a sense of purpose and fulfillment for a vibrant and fulfilling life: Ultimately, vitality is about more than just physical health—it's about leading a fulfilling and purposeful life. How can we cultivate a sense of purpose and fulfillment that contributes to our overall vitality? We'll explore the importance of meaningful activities, connections, and personal growth in our pursuit of lifelong well-being.

Conclusion

Congratulations on completing the journey through the secrets of a healthy life! We've covered a wealth of information on nutrition, fitness, mental and emotional well-being, healthy habits, relationships, environmental influences, preventive health measures, and the journey to lifelong vitality. As you reflect on this holistic approach to health and well-being, I encourage you to take the first steps towards a healthier, more vital life. Embrace the journey of lifelong wellness and vitality, and remember that every small, positive change you make can have a profound impact on your overall well-being. Here's to your vibrant and fulfilling life!

Ending Page

Dear Reader,

As you reach the final pages of "The Vitality Code," I extend my heartfelt gratitude for embarking on this transformative journey with me. Throughout these chapters, we've explored the intricate tapestry of health, happiness, and vitality, uncovering the profound connections between mind, body, and spirit. It has been my honor to be your guide, and I hope that the insights shared within these pages have ignited a spark of inspiration within you.

Remember, your journey to lifelong vitality is not a destination but a continuous evolution—a sacred dance between embracing the present moment and envisioning the possibilities of tomorrow. As you navigate the twists and turns of life, may you always hold fast to the belief that within you lies the power to thrive, to overcome, and to flourish in every season.

As you close this book, I encourage you to carry its wisdom with you as a beacon of hope and guidance on your path forward. Embrace the nourishing power of whole foods, the invigorating energy of movement, and the transformative magic of mindfulness. Cultivate gratitude, seek joy, and cherish the connections that enrich your life.

In the words of Rumi, "Live life as if everything is rigged in your favor." Trust in the innate wisdom of your body, the resilience of your spirit, and the boundless potential that resides within you. May you walk boldly, love fiercely, and live fully, embracing each moment with grace and gratitude.

With warmest wishes and deepest blessings,

Zohaib Hassan Khan

Wishing You Good Luck with Some Important Quotes:

"Health is the greatest gift, contentment the greatest wealth, faithfulness the best relationship." - Buddha

"The greatest wealth is health." - Virgil

"To keep the body in good health is a duty... otherwise we shall not be able to keep our mind strong and clear." - Buddha

"The groundwork of all happiness is health." - Leigh Hunt

"Your body holds deep wisdom. Trust in it. Learn from it. Nourish it. Watch your life transform and be healthy." - Bella Bleue

"Take care of your body. It's the only place you have to live." - Jim Rohn

"The first wealth is health." - Ralph Waldo Emerson

"Happiness is the highest form of health." - Dalai Lama

www.ingramcontent.com/pod-product-compliance
Lightning Source LLC
Chambersburg PA
CBHW070754250726
48662CB00004B/1807